Acupuncture

By: Erik Smith

Table Of Contents

Free Bonus!

Do Want To Master your fitness and health so you can feel and look amazing in the next 60 days?

I have a free bonus for you that can help dramatically improve your health in fitness that I think you will like. I have put together a 5-Day email course that will help you look amazing, but more importantly you will also feel great as well.

If that's something you think you would like, sign up to get the emails starting today.

Sign up here - https://enlightenedmanuals.com/5-health-steps/

Free Books Every Week!

Do you want to get notified when I have free books? Then sign up for my newsletter. I will never spam you. I will only send you valuable stuff that you can use to help you improve your life.

Sign up here - https://enlightenedmanuals.com/free-books/

Disclaimer

This document is geared towards providing exact and reliable information in regards to the topic and issue covered. The publication is sold with the idea that the publisher is not required to render accounting, officially permitted, or otherwise, qualified services. If advice is necessary, legal or professional, a practiced individual in the profession should be ordered.

- From a Declaration of Principles which was accepted and approved equally by a Committee of the American Bar Association and a Committee of Publishers and Associations.

The information herein is offered for informational purposes solely, and is universal as so. The presentation of the information is without contract or any type of guarantee assurance.

The trademarks that are used are without any consent, and the publication of the trademark is without permission or backing by the trademark owner. All trademarks and brands within this book are for clarifying purposes only and are the owned by the owners themselves, not affiliated with this document.

Introduction

Acupuncture is an ancient art that has been around for thousands of years. Although it is an established and regulated healing technique, many still think that it is shrouded with mystery.

Over the years, however, acupuncture has grown in popularity and the need for it has become more pronounced. In our modern times, too many people are getting caught up in the hustle and bustle of life. Health issues become more common, but the medications that are often most readily available end up having horrible side effects. Some of these medications are not even as effective as you are led to believe. Knowing all the possible options is a great help in finding the best medical technique, which can work for you.

Acupuncture has been tried and tested in many countries since the ancient times. This alternative Asian healing technique continues to bring relief and healing to people who suffer from many ailments. Discover and learn more about acupuncture as you delve deeper into this book.

Fundamentals of Acupuncture

Acupuncture is one of the oldest and most widely known forms of Chinese therapy. It is likely that you have seen this form of therapy featured on television or on the internet and there many people who swear by its positive effects. Still, it remains a mystery for the general public.

If you have seen acupuncture being done then it's fairly certain that you have plenty of questions in mind. This is especially true because acupuncture is such a far cry from the allopathic western medicine that you're probably used to. What is acupuncture and how does it work? In this chapter, you will be introduced to acupuncture, the ancient philosophies that produced this ancient technique, as well as some modern takes on this subject.

Basics

The word acupuncture comes from combining two Latin words Acus, meaning needle, and puncture, which means to puncture. Acupuncture is a minimally invasive therapeutic technique. An acupuncturist will have to place fine needles into certain points of your body as a means of healing and stimulating them whether for overall health, or for specific conditions, such as diabetes, high blood pressure, etc.

More advanced practices use heat, magnets and electricity along with the needles. Some techniques don't use needles, at all. Instead, they simply use magnets with mild electrical currents to stimulate the acupressure points.

How exactly does placing needles and using magnets and electricity on the body help you heal?

Ancient thought behind acupuncture

Acupuncture has a rich tradition and philosophy behind it dating back thousands of years and despite negative associations from the medical industry, it continues to grow and thrive.

Chinese medicine, acupuncture in particular, operates around the central concept of the Qi, or the energy that is in every living being. This can be translated as life force, or life energy, which brings life to all beings. This life energy flows through every organ, limb and cell of the body through meridians or channels.

Not a comparison

If you want to understand acupuncture and its functions, you have to realize that you cannot compare it to Western medicine, and you have to put aside your scientific view of anatomy. Keep in mind that the philosophies behind acupuncture and traditional Chinese Medicine were formulated before any scientific advancement in anatomy and physiology, not to mention the wholly different views regarding health and well-being.

When the lung meridian or the Qi channel responsible for the lungs is mentioned, do not expect it to be anywhere near where the lungs are. Acupuncture is more about healing an aspect of the human body, which is beyond just the physical.

Balance and Flow of Energy

In acupuncture, your good health is maintained when there is unhindered flow and balance in the Qi or life force through the channels, as well as having good circulation of blood, lymph and other bodily fluids. When these channels get clogged up or if there is too much or too little energy, then you get sick.

The channels all throughout your body carry Qi and each channel is responsible for a certain organ and function. These channels, in turn, have certain points with varying yet related functions when stimulated by acupuncture needles.

The food you eat, excesses of any kind and even your own emotions can have positive or negative effects on the flow of qi and the energy balance in your body. By stimulating these points with the acupuncture needles, an acupuncturist can strengthen your qi and balance your energies.

The Concept of Yin and Yang

It is almost absolutely certain that everyone has, at some point, seen the symbol for yin and yang. If you think you haven't, you probably have and you just didn't know what it stood for.

For those who are unfamiliar, the symbol for yin and yang is a circle, which is divided into black and white, but not straight down the middle. They are converging towards each other, and on the white half of the circle is a small black dot, and vice versa on the black half. The yin and yang symbol is popular in pop culture but what does it mean?

The concept of yin and yang is actually a simplistic view of dialectics, or the belief that it is possible to divide any object into two seemingly opposing forces. Yin and yang is about the merging and oneness of opposites, such as dark and light, cold and hot, male and female, that are contrasting and contradicting each other, thus, bringing life and change. Additionally, it is also about transformation, which is why there is a black dot in the white part and vice versa. This means that these elements can transform and change into each other as well, and that one cannot exist without the other.

The main example ancient Chinese scholars had of these contradicting properties was fire and water. Yin stood for everything that can be likened to or simulates the characteristics of water, i.e. it is cold, flows downward, dim or has an element of darkness. On the other hand, Yang stood for the properties of fire, i.e. it is hot, it billows upwards and it is bright.

In relation to acupuncture, the points, channels, the organs and their functions within the body are also divided by their Yin and Yang characteristics. Every organ must work accordingly or else there will be an imbalance in the Yin and Yang energies. For example, Yin functions can get too strong and weaken the Yang and vice versa, or a certain channel may get clogged up and bring about an excess, or a deficiency, in a certain aspect.

When imbalances like these occur, an acupuncturist will then stimulate points that strengthen or regulate that Yin or Yang organ, thereby restoring the balance of energy in your body.

A modern take on Acupuncture

Since acupuncture has changed so many lives and now has millions of people, even in the West, who are swearing by it, the scientific community can't just disregard the benefits. You can see this through the advent of

licensed acupuncturists even in the West and of doctors with medical degrees taking advanced courses in acupuncture.

Scientists have worked hard to try and explain how and why it works on a more materialistic and scientific level and there have been some interesting findings.

Bioelectrical Energy

In the 1950's, scientists noticed that there were electrical properties in the skin along the channels and points that differed from areas of the skin without points or channels. Scientists also found that this electrical potential was affected when an organ was damaged or removed or if the channel's path was blocked by damaged tissues. Many practitioners believe that it is this electrical connection between the channels and the organs they govern that is at the heart of acupuncture.

Biomagnetism

Acupuncture practitioners were able to demonstrate a relationship between the qi channels and the natural magnetic fields in the body. By placing bio magnets on acupuncture points, they were able to measure certain nervous micro-currents found in the nerves that affected blood flow.

Chinese medicine, along with acupuncture, moxibustion, and acupressure, differs greatly from western medicine in the sense that instead of fixing just one aspect (by drinking medicine specifically designed for it) or by replacing a certain organ when it gives up, it tries to bring balance to the body as a whole. Instead of just replacing parts, as in an engine, you are getting a full tune-up. Even if you may be exploring acupuncture to fix a certain specific problem, your entire body can benefit and the positive effects can even surprise you.

The History and Evolution of Acupuncture

Acupuncture and its brothers in Chinese medicine come from a deep well of medical knowledge that not only endured, but even flourished for thousands of years. It is not just China. Many Asian countries, such as Japan and India, have also brought on their own influences in this collective knowledge, and the practice continues to improve and evolve today.

In this chapter, you will explore the fascinating and vast history of acupuncture that began more than three thousand years ago.

Ancient Roots

In the olden days, when there was no knowledge of viruses and bacteria, those in the medical field would simply observe nature and its effects on people. Why, for example, do people get sick more often during cold, monsoon seasons? Or why do people get headaches when the sun was too hot.

'Natural' beginnings

Nature ended up becoming a dominant factor when it comes to Chinese medicine and regions with varying climates played different roles in the development of the practice.

For example, in the cold northern region of China where flora was limited to bushes and grasses, they practiced placing dried mugwort, a type of grass, which grows in the cold climate, on certain points of the body and setting it on fire. The heat, placed in specific acu-points, could bring about much needed relief from the extremely cold temperature of the region.

Similarly, the medical practice in the southern region, where land was fertile and the weather was warm, involved the use of herbs, barks and roots that were in abundance. This convergence of knowledge has become a basis for Chinese herbal remedies.

Old and extensive

Evidence of acupuncture and its practice was found as early as 1000 B.C. when archeologists found acupuncture needles and information carved into bones that dated from the ancient Shang Dynasty. Through trade and travel, northern and southern knowledge began to combine and, by 400 A.D., a rather sophisticated medical practice grew in China.

This much needed and advanced (for its time) medical knowledge spread throughout East Asian Countries. As this medical practice and theory was applied in different places, with a different set of medical problems to deal with, the practice grew and evolved. Different customs, beliefs and practical knowledge accumulated as time passed.

Acupuncture through Cultures

Because acupuncture has passed through so many cultures for such a long time, it is normal that there are many different interpretations and practical knowledge surrounding it. Different cultures have all left their own unique stamp on acupuncture.

Traditional Chinese Medicine

This is the main branch of acupuncture and follows the 3000 year old teachings of the Ancient Chinese practice. This practice involves the concept of balancing the yin and yang. The famous bronze man proves the Ancient

Chinese's desire to learn and unlock the secrets of medicine.

The bronze man was a small bronze statue that was used to train students who were learning acupuncture. It helped familiarize them with the placement of the points as well as the depth and angle of needling. The bronze man is still used by modern practitioners, but instead of being made of bronze, it is now made of soft plastic.

The Five Elements Theory

This is an additional body of knowledge and philosophy that was incorporated to TCM at around 400 B.C. It is the concept that all things are made of vital elements namely, wood, fire, earth and water. You can even see this concept being carried over to the Chinese zodiac.

Your body, personality and even your ailments are governed and are changed by the relationships between these elements. Certain excesses and emotional distress are also attributed to imbalances between the elements.

This still falls into the yin and yang philosophy as elements can often be found together, with varying elements being dominant in a certain person. Also, the different elements react with each other in a rather dialectical way, through promotion, suppression, action and counter-action. For example, water promotes wood, which in turn promotes fire, while water suppresses fire; wood suppresses earth, which then suppresses water.

Japanese Acupuncture

The principles of TCM were also adapted by the Japanese, but they have taken it a step further and developed their own particular additions to the method of diagnosis and treatment. The body "map" of channels that go through the body is still used, but with farther insight and a more composed usage of the points.

A certain Japanese method of diagnosis involves the hara, identified with the abdomen and called the sea of qi. Subsequent palpations around this area are believed to reveal problems in your health.

Another particular aspect of Japanese Acupuncture is the use of your own body's magnetic field in healing and adjusting the balance of Qi and energy.

Acupuncture in the Western World

Because of the need and interest to find alternative ways to stay healthy and find balance in the high-strung, fast-paced modern world, Acupuncture has found resurgence in the west. Conventional allopathic medicine or mainstream western medicine has started to give leeway and even merge with the ancient and proven arts of Eastern medicine.

Several states in the US have now passed regulations regarding acupuncture, and there are even acupuncture schools and courses being taught in several colleges. In many states, the acupuncture course is a 3-year master's degree, which requires a bachelor of premed courses.

It is safe to say that acupuncture is now being treated as a true science. Of course, there are still many critics who question the validity of this method and the scientific basis for it, but there is so much about the human body, which still remains a mystery. The results speak for themselves. Cases and testimonials of people whose lives were changed by acupuncture continue to grow, adding to acupuncture's relevance in the modern world.

The Possibilities of Acupuncture

Acupuncture holds many possibilities for proponents of alternative medicine. There have been many people at the end of their ropes who found hope in the practice. There are countless of testimonials coming from people who have tried every medication and western therapy style they could without any improvements in their condition. They have only found sweet relief through acupuncture.

There are many ailments that acupuncture can definitely help with, but keep in mind that you cannot use it exclusively to cure all ailments. It is, however, possible for you to use it in conjunction with medication as long as you consult your doctor and your acupuncture practitioner about it.

Acupuncture Efficacy

According to ancient Chinese teachings and some modern practitioners, there are points for nearly every ailment, from diabetes to cholera, to cancer and the common cold. There are acupuncture points for every disease conceivable.

However, it is important to note that acupuncture aims to strengthen YOU and not defeat or destroy the disease. It is part of the Naturopathic way of healing, where the body is healed without introducing any chemicals or substances. Instead, you are being healed from the inside. By fixing up your own energy levels, your body is more capable of healing itself.

Unlike medications like antibiotics that target the bacteria causing the sickness itself, acupuncture aims to make your resistance against bacteria stronger. Acupuncture strengthens your body, making it capable to defeat the disease itself.

This, in itself, is already a good thing for you, but when it comes to serious infections that require immediate action, acupuncture alone may not provide the needed relief. Nevertheless, it offers many possibilities.

Acupuncture works great on:

·   Pain management – Even detractors of acupuncture have to admit that it helps people manage pain, although some attribute it to the placebo effect. What detractors can't explain, however, is why certain people who have tried the strongest pain meds available stand by acupuncture.

Pain meds often target nervous centers in the brain to keep someone from feeling pain, but despite this, patients still often feel pain along with the corresponding nasty side effects. All this is cut out when they choose to undergo acupuncture.

·   Any issues related to the nervous system – Acupuncture does wonders for nervous system problems. All forms of paralysis, migraines, insomnia, and all forms of neuralgia respond well with acupuncture therapy. In acupuncture, pain is considered as a blockage in the Qi channel and is in line with clearing passages.

·   Digestive and respiratory problems – Acupuncture has proven to be effective in treating disorders in the digestive and respiratory system, such as ulcers, diarrhea, vomiting, acidity, asthma, dry cough, and tonsillitis.

·   Mental and psychological disorders – There are acupuncture points and combinations that can treat psychological disorders.

·   Sexual and urological disorders – Urinary pain, dysfunction in the urological system as well as problems with sexual fertility, impotence and other problems in the reproductive system have shown to respond well to the therapy.

·   Eyes, skin and hair issues

Acupuncture Risks

Yes, there are definitely some risks when it comes to acupuncture, but every form of medication has risks. The risks in acupuncture, however, are really small and can easily be avoided by experienced practitioners.

In Japan and China, places where there are millions of treatments being done every year, there have only been 10 injuries reported since 1972. The numbers in the U.S. correspond to this number with 10 reported injuries since 1965. This is a far cry from the millions of injuries and negative side effects caused by conventional procedures and allopathic drugs.

Risk factors and the (easy) solutions

·   Bleeding – This is normal and can happen since needles are breaking the skin. Just put pressure on the point.

·   Infection from a dirty needle – Just make sure that your practitioner is licensed and is using brand new needles.

·   Pain because of a blunt needle – This is easily remedied by new needles.

·   Anxiousness of the patient – Just close your eyes and relax.

Counter indications

·   Skin ulcers, eczema and burns should not be punctured. Not only is the spot sore but dirt from the surface of the skin can go inside and worsen infection.

·   Nipples and fatty tissue of the breast. There are no acupuncture points in this area and the area is also very sensitive.

·   Main arteries and veins. Accidentally puncturing a blood vessel can cause bruising, but an experienced acupuncturist can work easily around this.

·   Pregnancy. Although there are certain points that are safe for pregnant women, most points on the lower body are counter indicated.

It is important to recognize the actual possibilities as well as certain limitations that acupuncture has. Make sure to get a balanced medical plan and strategy by talking to your doctor and therapist.

Before Treatment - Acupuncture Diagnosis

Now that you know the history of acupuncture and the immensely rich body of knowledge from which it sprang, you are thinking about having your first session. Still, fear may creep into your mind. How is it going to feel?

Will there be blood since you'll be stuck with needles after all? Is it completely safe?

Not to worry, reign in your fears and allow yourself to be surprised and even amazed at how simple, painless and safe acupuncture actually is. This chapter is going to be about putting your fears to rest and going into your first session with relaxed confidence.

Diagnosis, simple yet effective

Acupuncture diagnosis is simple and easy, but it actually takes an experienced eye to see the nuances. Unlike allopathic medicine, which treats specific symptoms and ailments and is therefore based on specific, often expensive tests, an acupuncture practitioner will simply diagnose the balances and imbalances through your general appearance, a tongue and pulse diagnosis, and the physical symptoms you feel.

The power of observation: Your general appearance

Your chosen practitioner will first look at you as a whole. They will note your posture, the tone and texture of your skin, your expression and even your weight. All these aspects are affected by your overall health and the balance of qi energy in your body.

For example, being overweight can mean a weakness in Yang energy, which has to do with being active and burning energy, along with some excesses in dampness, which slows down circulation and can lead to lethargy.

Having pale skin and dark lines under the eyes can mean weak blood circulation and deficiencies found in or around the kidney and spleen channels. On the other hand, having a flushed face and an overly thin body type can mean an excess in heat and, either weakness of the yin energy, or over action of yang organs.

There are many interpretations and possible diagnoses. This general observation diagnosis is going to see how your body is in general, then will be related to the current symptoms and the findings of your tongues diagnosis.

The secrets in your tongue

According to Oriental medicine, any aspect of the body has its counterpart in the tongue. The health and balance of every channel and organ can be seen by examining the tongue. It can seem as if all tongues are the same, but this is not true at all.

Take a moment to look at your tongue in the mirror and notice the little peculiarities. Do you notice little red bumps that are evident on the surface of your tongue? Take a note of the size, overall shape and color of your tongue and the fuzzy coating or film, which is usually colored white or yellow. You may even notice some cracks and bumps in certain areas. Believe it or not, all of these factor in on your diagnosis.

For example, a thin tongue with a bright red tip can mean a lot of emotional upheaval or stimulation. This can also mean a lot of heat in your heart.

Once your acupuncture practitioner has made the necessary observation, he or she will talk to you about the findings. This is actually an important aspect of the whole diagnosis process since finding out your lifestyle, general emotional disposition, and discomforts you may feel in your body also offers important insights into the energy flow and imbalances in your body. Do you remember yin and yang and the five elements? Well emotions fall into these categories as well.

Pulse Diagnosis

The power of the pulse to tell more about the inner workings of your own body is lost in modern science, but this is a subtle and important aspect of diagnosis. A trained practitioner can distinguish depths and pulse positions that give great insight into your overall health. The diagnosis is based on three pulse positions that run along the area of your wrist.

The strength, general feel and depth of your pulse all indicate certain traits surrounding your current health. For example, a slow or weak pulse on the middle position can mean trapped coldness within the body, while a slippery feel to your pulse, which means instead of a strong beat, it feels like thick, squishy liquid under the fingers, can mean a disruption caused by excess dampness.

A practitioner will generally do an overall observation and either a tongue or a pulse diagnosis. He will then discuss the findings as well as the channels and corresponding organs he or she will be working on. You will also talk about the frequency through which you will need to undergo treatments and your next treatment schedule.

If you find that your practitioner is using terminology that you can't understand, all you have to do is ask. If you are interested, you can also ask about the specific points that he intends to use, as well as the corresponding function of each. It is your body after all.

The Treatment

Now that you and your practitioner have a general agreement about what is wrong, how many needles have to be used and where, it is time to go under the needle. The treatment is often done in a private and quiet area. You will probably be made to lie down on a massage table or sit on a chair, depending on the points needed to be reached.

Relax and breathe

Once you are suitably positioned and ready, then the needle insertions can begin. Most acupuncturists will use needles only once for a particular patient. Although there are reusable needles, it should only be reusable for the person it was used on and not on anyone else. You will find, however, that most acupuncturists will always use new needles.

The acupuncture practitioner will do his or her utmost to help you relax, inviting you to breathe or letting you listen to music if needed. Relaxation is important, since stress can cause your muscles to contract and make it harder for the needle to be inserted smoothly.

Will it hurt?

Now for the million dollar question, will having needles inserted into your skin without any local or general anesthetic hurt? The truth, surprisingly, is no. The insertion of the needle itself is quick and rather painless. There are many instances when people don't even notice that the needles have already been placed.

There are, however, instances when you do feel something. This greatly depends on the particular skill, style as well as the thickness of the needles used (there are needles that are especially fine while there are thicker and sturdier ones). Although you may feel a prick, it never lasts long and can hardly be considered a painful experience.

If you ever had your ears pierced then you would have no problem with acupuncture, which is by far less painful.

Finding the points: Proportional measurements

The general location of all the points in the body are the same for every person, but having a universal measuring system won't work for every body type. This is why the point measurement in acupuncture is proportional.

Instead of using a universal unit of measurement, your points are found through the proportional measurements of your own fingers.

The distance of the creases of the interphalangeal joints (or the second to the last joint up to the last joint) of the middle finger, as well as the width of the last joint in your thumb is considered one cun. The width of your four fingers (without the thumb) is three cun.

You can measure your points in accordance to your own fingers, so expect your acupuncture practitioner to measure your hands and fingers against theirs before finding your points.

The session

Depending on the points used, the acupuncturist will typically leave the needles in for 20 minutes to an hour. Every point has its own particular angling and depth of insertion to hit the point, with some needles being shorter and just going a little deeper than the skin, and others being longer, going down to about an inch or more, depending on the area.

Of course, insertion depth and placement will depend on your proportional measurements. For example, a shallow insertion may not do for a bigger person, while going too deep on a skinny person can cause the needle to go over the mark.

During the entirety of the session, you will be expected to lay still. After all, there are needles inside your skin. These can get bent if you move or suddenly change your position. Don't worry though, as your acupuncturist will be present to keep a close eye on you.

A tingling sensation

It has already been established that needling itself does not hurt, but what sensations can you expect once the session is underway? Typical sensations felt during acupuncture treatment can include tingling, an almost electrical "buzz", and a dull ache, or numbness. Some people have described it as having a stack of books laid over the points. This can be attributed to the stimulation of the qi energy in the points.

Remember to stay relaxed. Acupuncture can even be considered as an almost meditative experience, as you become more aware and focused on the sensations of the body.

After Treatment

Depending on the diagnosis, there can be certain restrictions for you after acupuncture. The universal restriction, however, is not getting the puncture point wet or dirty 2 hours after the session. This is a simple precaution so that the punctured points do not get infected. An hour or two gives your body ample time to close up the puncture points since the needles used are extremely fine.

Other restrictions can include heavy, calorie laden, meals or big meat dishes, extreme exercise, or excessive alcohol intake 12-24 hours after the session. These can be counterproductive to the acupuncture treatment or can cause an inverse reaction so soon after treatment.

Where to get acupuncture sessions

The simplest, easiest and safest way to find acupuncture practitioners and professionals is by connecting to organizations that certify the profession. There are many online organizations with records of skilled and certified acupuncture practitioners. Make sure to visit a practitioner with the right credentials and is known to be a true professional.

Now that you know that acupuncture is being performed by well regulated and educated professionals, and is a safe and established art, what can stop you from having you first session? Acupuncture may just be the kind of therapy you need.

Conclusion

Thank you for downloading this eBook! Hopefully this book was able to reveal the secrets of acupuncture to you and help you understand this ancient and time-tested technique.

Don't think you're done though. There are still so many things about acupuncture that you have to learn. The best thing to do is to go out and have your first session with a licensed and experienced practitioner. Don't forget to tell your family about it afterwards as well. Thank you and good health!

Free Bonus!

Do Want To Master your fitness and health so you can feel and look amazing in the next 60 days?

I have a free bonus for you that can help dramatically improve your health in fitness that I think you will like. I have put together a 5-Day email course that will help you look amazing, but more importantly you will also feel great as well.

If that's something you think you would like, sign up to get the emails starting today.

Sign up here - https://enlightenedmanuals.com/5-health-steps/

Free Books Every Week!

Do you want to get notified when I have free books? Then sign up for my newsletter. I will never spam you. I will only send you valuable stuff that you can use to help you improve your life.

Sign up here - https://enlightenedmanuals.com/free-books/

www.ingramcontent.com/pod-product-compliance
Lightning Source LLC
Chambersburg PA
CBHW050527290526
45786CB00007B/2732